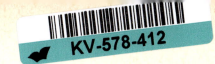

612-399

This book is to be returned on or before
the last date stamped below.

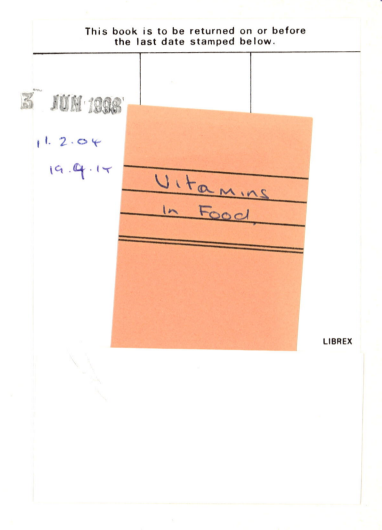

Vitamins
In Food,

LIBREX

DIET AND NUTRITION

Vitamins in Food

Miriam Moss

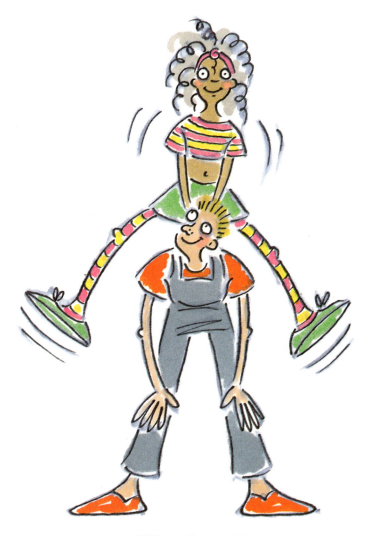

Wayland

DIET AND NUTRITION

Additives in Food
Vitamins in Food
Fibre in Food
Sugar in Food

Series Editor: Deborah Elliott
Designer: Malcolm Walker
Cover design: Simon Balley
Artwork: John Yates
Cartoons: Maureen Jackson

First published in 1995 by
Wayland (Publishers) Limited
61 Western Road, Hove,
East Sussex, BN3 1JD, England

Text is based on *Vitamins* in the *Food Facts* series,
published in 1992

British Library Cataloguing in Publication Data
Moss. Miriam
 Vitamins in food - (Diet and Nutrition series)
 I. Title   II. Series
 612.399

 ISBN 0 7502 1436 8

Typesetting by Kudos Editorial and Design Services
Printed and bound by Rotolito Lombarda s.p.a. Italy

Contents

Staying healthy

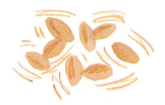

Your body is like a machine. It needs food for energy, just like a car needs fuel to run. As well as giving you energy, the food you eat contains vitamins and minerals. Your body needs these vitamins and minerals to help you grow and to stay healthy.

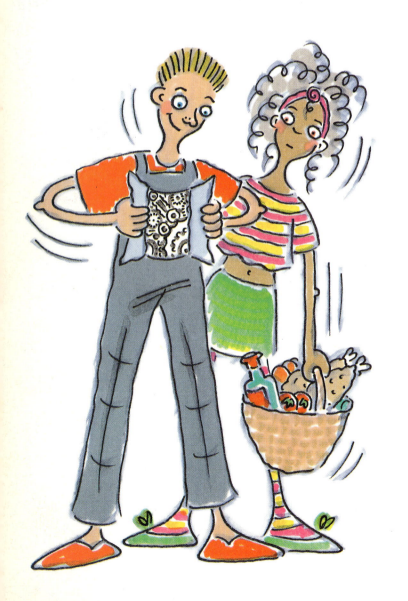

▶ *Can you see the rice seeds flying through the air on the opposite page? These farmers are threshing rice stalks so that the seeds fall into a huge pile at their feet. The outside husks of rice are full of a vitamin called B1.*

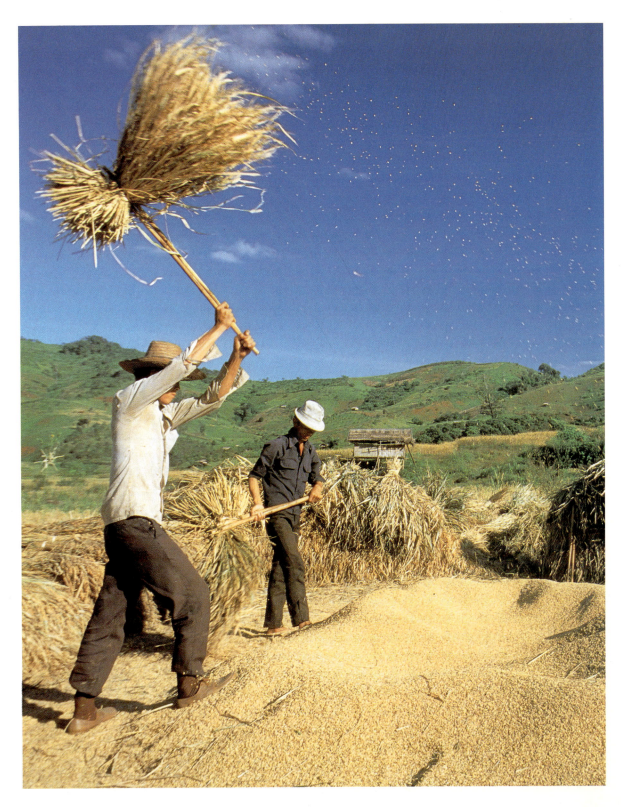

Fruit for life

Long ago sailors went on sea voyages and didn't eat any fruit or vegetables for many weeks. Often they caught a horrible disease called scurvy, which caused sore gums and bleeding under the skin. Soon doctors realized that sailors who ate lemons and limes didn't get scurvy.

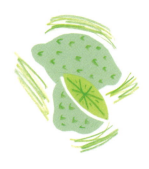

▼ *The important vitamin in citrus fruits, like these unripe lemons, is called vitamin C.*

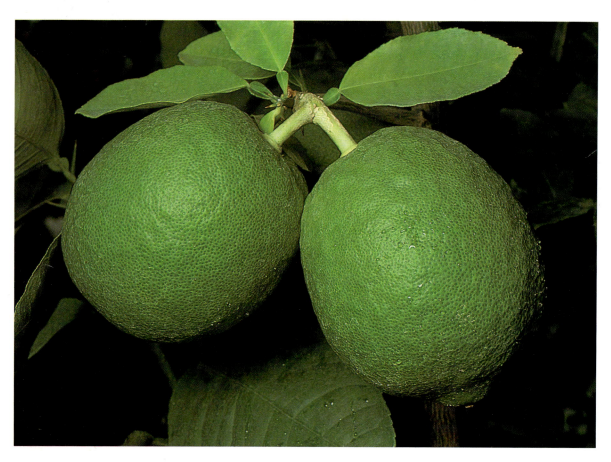

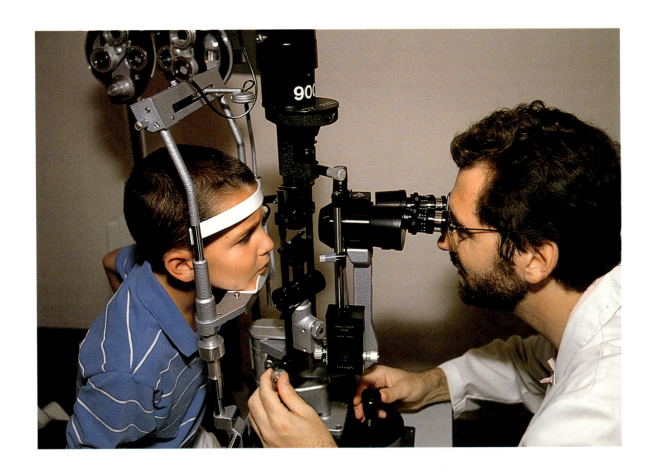

This boy is having his eyes tested. The vitamin which helps keep your eyes healthy is vitamin A. It is found in egg yokes and in butter. In Greek and Roman times, people knew that if they ate liver and cod-liver oil it helped to stop them getting an illness called night blindness. Night blindness means that you cannot see anything at all in the dark.

► *These pills contain vitamins. Always remember to check with an adult before taking a pill.*

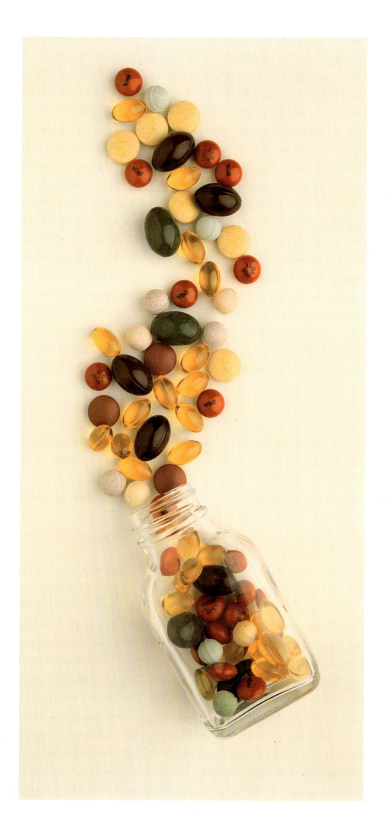

One by one, the vitamins we know about today were discovered. Each vitamin was named after a letter of the alphabet.

The boy in the photograph is taking a spoonful of cod-liver oil, which is rich in vitamin D. Vitamin D was discovered because doctors noticed that children living in countries with lots of sunshine did not get a disease called rickets.

Rickets softens the bones so that leg bones, for example, become bent. Vitamin D is found in sunlight and in cod-liver oil.

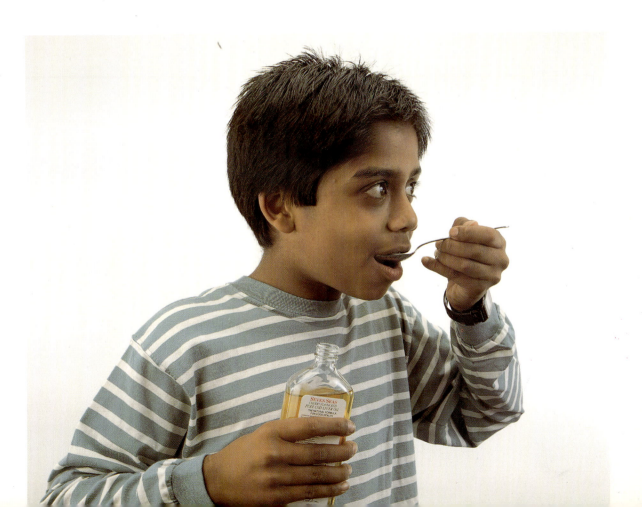

Vitamin A
for your eyes!

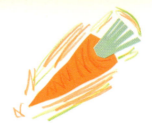

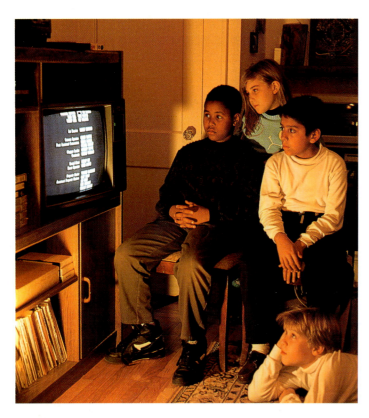

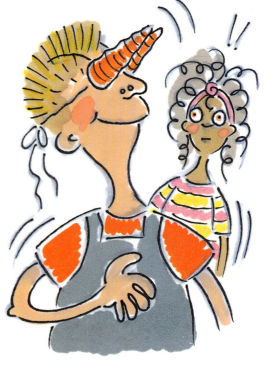

Question: Is it true that eating carrots helps you to see in the dark?

Answer: Yes! Carrots contain a yellow colouring called carotene which is rich in vitamin A.

Watching television in a dark room uses up a lot of vitamin A.

Vitamins with special names

Food wrappings, such as cereal packets, show which vitamins the food contains. Some vitamins have special names. Folic acid belongs to the group of B vitamins. Look for some of the specially named vitamins on this chart. Copy the chart and then write down where you find these vitamins.

	Ascorbic acid	Folic acid	Niacin	Riboflavin	Thiamin
	(Vit C)	(B Group)	(B Group)	(B Group)	(B Group)
Where it is found	lemon barley water		Cornflakes	Cornflakes	Cornflakes

Vitamin A is in most dark green or yellow fruit and vegetables, such as parsley, marrows, apricots, oranges, peaches and melons. It is also in fish-liver oils, milk and butter. Vitamin A helps to make strong bones and teeth and it helps us to recover from illnesses faster.

B vitamins stay cool

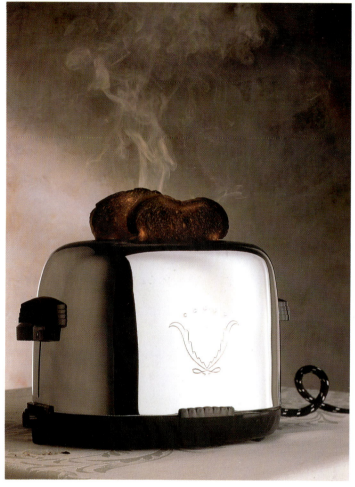

► *A lot of the vitamin B in bread is lost when toast is burnt.* ✓

B vitamins need to stay cool, because they are easily damaged by heat. Up to half the B vitamins in food are destroyed by cooking.

There are thirteen kinds of B vitamins. They look after our brains, our skin and the way we digest food. B vitamins are found in milk, wheat germ, liver, cereals and yeast.

Eating green leafy vegetables is very good for you because they contain folic acid. Folic acid is a very important B vitamin which is needed to make your blood and to keep your brain healthy.

Grow your own beans
Bean shoots are delicious and full of vitamins, so why not grow some yourself?
You will need: half a cup full of mung beans
                a jam jar and cover
                water
1.   Soak the beans in water overnight.
2.   Drain off the water and put the beans in the covered jam jar in a warm dark place.
3.   Rinse and drain the beans twice a day with warm water.
4.   After a few days, when the shoots are 5 cm long, eat them!

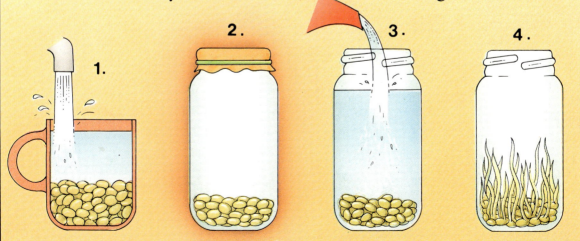

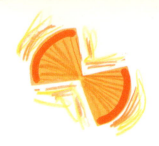

Vitamin C the healer!

Vitamin C helps to heal cuts, bruises and burns and it helps with healthy teeth and gums, blood and bones. You use up lots of vitamin C when you fight illnesses. As our bodies cannot store vitamin C, it is important to eat some food which is rich in vitamin C each day. Vitamin C comes in citrus fruits, green peppers and tomatoes.

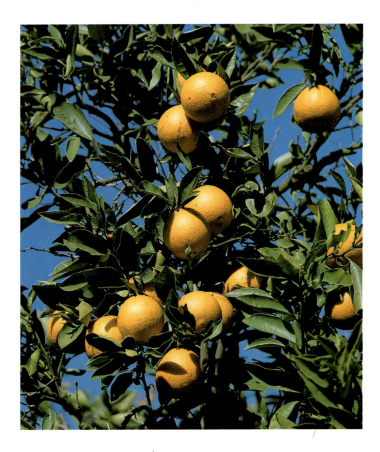

◀ *Oranges are full of vitamin C.*

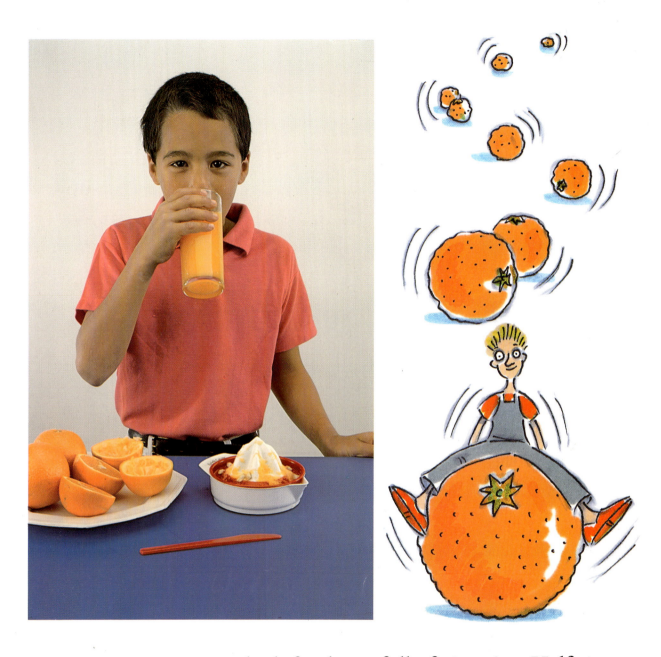

It is not easy to guess which foods are full of vitamins. Half a cupful of fresh bean sprouts contains as much vitamin C as six glasses of orange juice!

Real lemon drink

Many of the vitamins in the fruit drinks you buy have been destroyed. Try making your own fresh lemon drink full of vitamin C. (Get an adult to help you.)

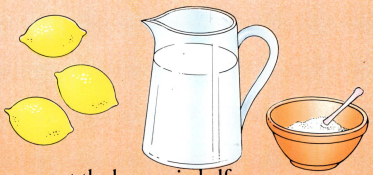

You will need:
4 fresh lemons
$^3/_4$ litre of hot water
sugar to taste

1. Ask an adult to help you cut the lemons in half.
2. Squeeze the juice into a jug.
3. Dissolve a little sugar in some hot water.
4. Add it to the lemon juice and mix them together.
5. Cool the lemon juice in the fridge for an hour. Then drink it!

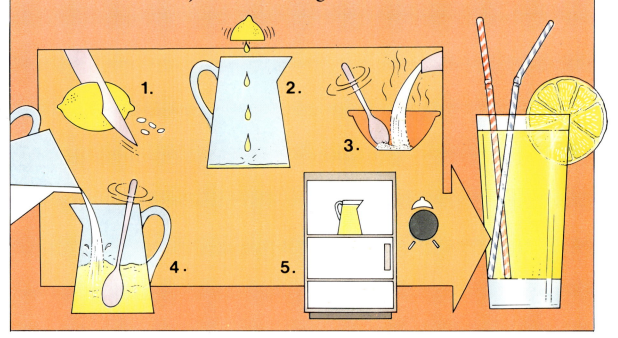

Sunny vitamin D

Vitamin D is called the sunny vitamin, because we get it from sunlight. Vitamin D is made when the sun shines on the oils found on our bare skin. People who live in countries with little sunlight might not get enough vitamin D. They may need to take vitamin D pills.

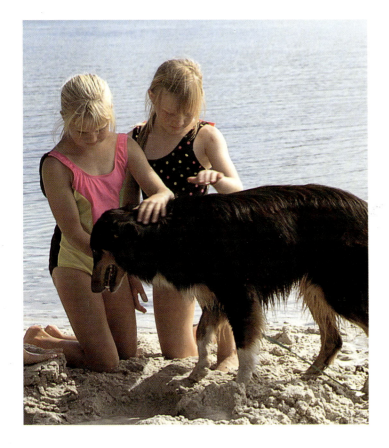

◀ *Remember not to stay out in the hot sun for too long, as sunshine can harm your skin.*

Miraculous vitamin E?

Vitamin E has become famous as a miracle cure for all sorts of things. Some say that it can make wrinkles fade and make a person look young for ever! Vitamin E does help to heal burns and scars, and it protects our lungs from air pollution. It also helps us to store vitamin A in our bodies longer.

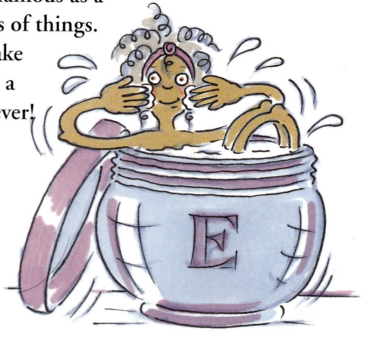

◀ *Vitamin E cream helps to cure dry skin.*

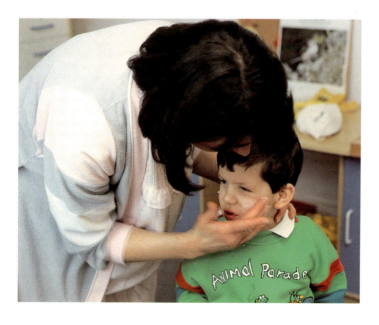

Check it out!

You can tell if you are getting enough of the five main vitamins on this chart by the way you look. Are your nails strong, your teeth healthy and your hair shiny?

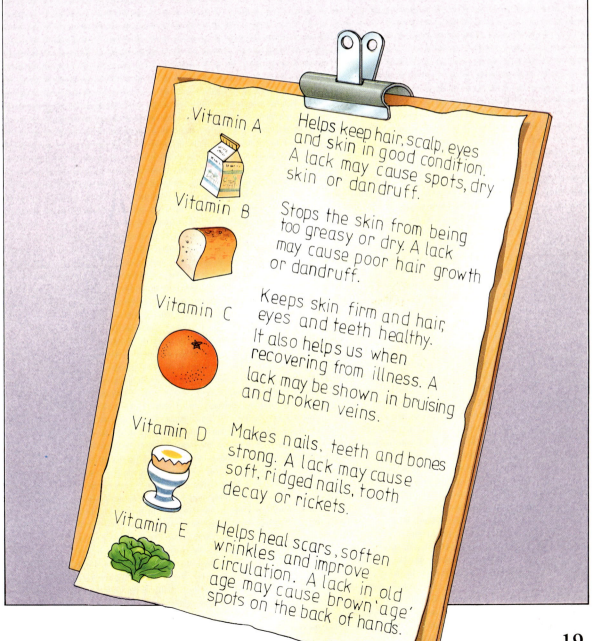

Vitamin A — Helps keep hair, scalp, eyes and skin in good condition. A lack may cause spots, dry skin or dandruff.

Vitamin B — Stops the skin from being too greasy or dry. A lack may cause poor hair growth or dandruff.

Vitamin C — Keeps skin firm and hair, eyes and teeth healthy. It also helps us when recovering from illness. A lack may be shown in bruising and broken veins.

Vitamin D — Makes nails, teeth and bones strong. A lack may cause soft, ridged nails, tooth decay or rickets.

Vitamin E — Helps heal scars, soften wrinkles and improve circulation. A lack in old age may cause brown 'age' spots on the back of hands.

MORE vitamins?

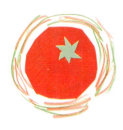

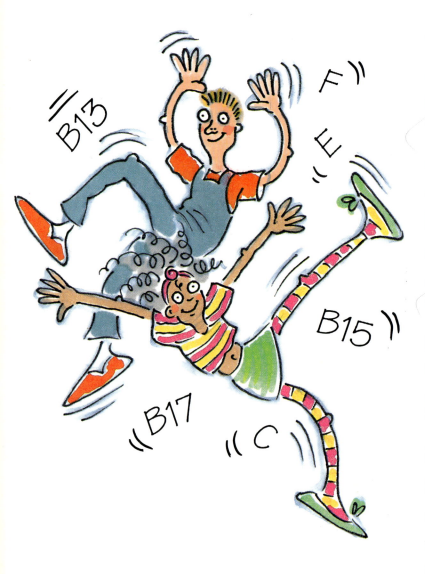

We have talked about the five main vitamins, but there are lots more! Vitamin P is found in the pulp and the pith of fruit. Vitamin K helps our blood to make scabs when we cut ourselves.

Vitamin K is found in green vegetables, tomatoes, honey, egg yolks and bran.

Vitamin B17 is found in the seeds of most fruits. Scientists keep discovering new vitamins. They try to find out as much about them as they can.

As well as vitamins, we also need minerals to stay healthy. Without minerals, our bodies cannot use vitamins. Calcium is the mineral which helps to keep our teeth strong. Regular brushing helps, too!

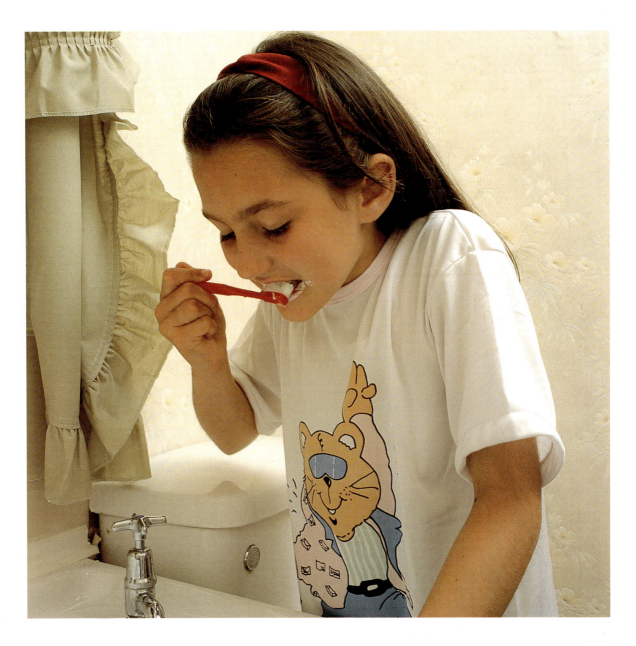

Five important minerals

Make a list of all the food and drinks you have had today. Look at this chart under the 'where to find them' column, to see which minerals your food or drinks contained. Have you had each of these five minerals today?

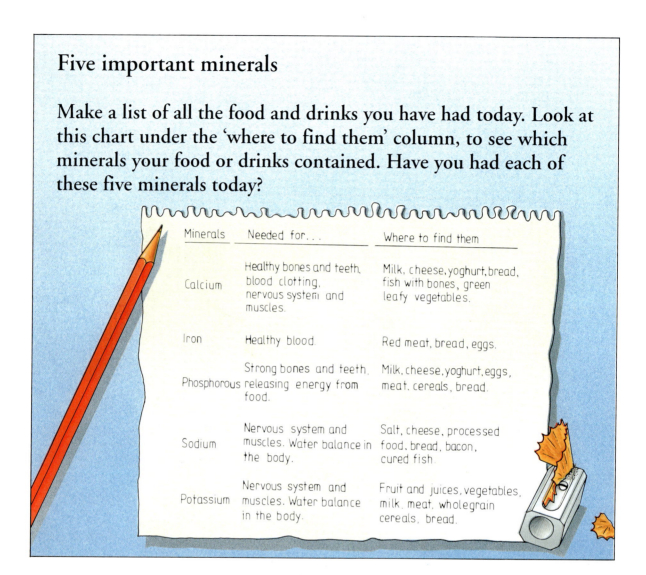

Minerals	Needed for...	Where to find them
Calcium	Healthy bones and teeth, blood clotting, nervous system and muscles.	Milk, cheese, yoghurt, bread, fish with bones, green leafy vegetables.
Iron	Healthy blood.	Red meat, bread, eggs.
Phosphorous	Strong bones and teeth, releasing energy from food.	Milk, cheese, yoghurt, eggs, meat, cereals, bread.
Sodium	Nervous system and muscles. Water balance in the body.	Salt, cheese, processed food, bread, bacon, cured fish.
Potassium	Nervous system and muscles. Water balance in the body.	Fruit and juices, vegetables, milk, meat, wholegrain cereals, bread.

Our bodies cannot make minerals, so we need to have a good supply from our food. Did you know that inside your body there is enough iron to make a 5 cm-long nail?

Pills, powders and liquids

One way of getting enough vitamins and minerals is to eat a healthy, balanced diet. If this is not possible, chemists sell pills, powders and liquids which have the right vitamins and minerals in them. Some of the vitamins and minerals are made from chemicals, and others are taken from plants and animals.

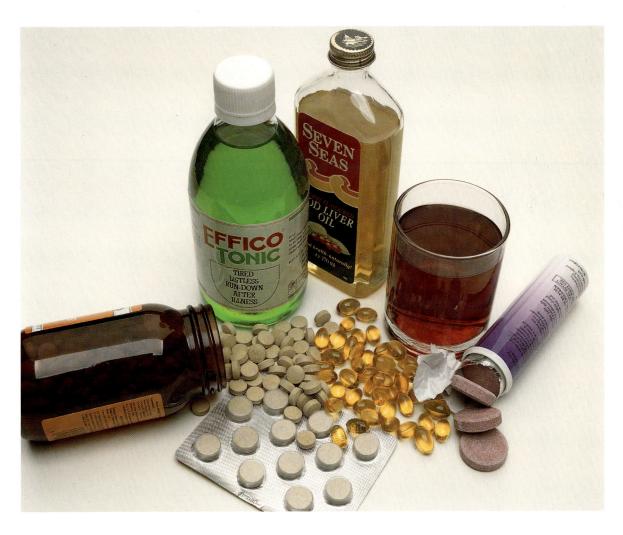

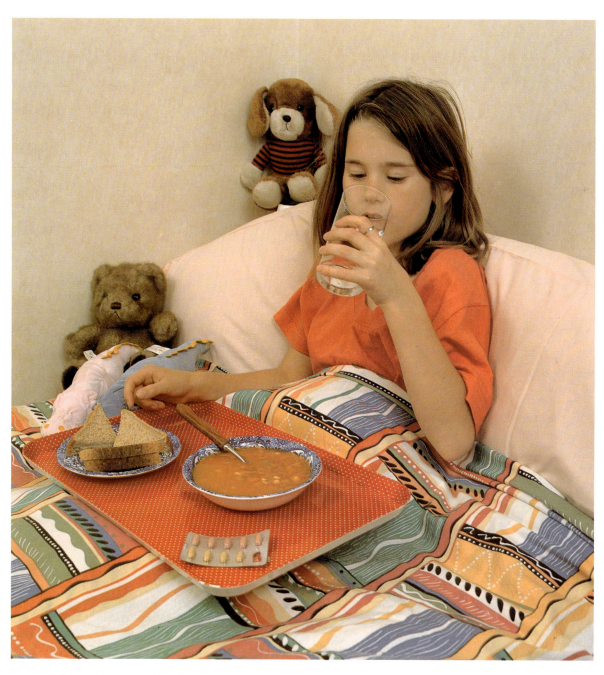

▲ *Vitamin and mineral pills can be useful when you are ill and don't feel like eating certain foods. They help you to get well again.*

There is a lot of disagreement about the amount of each vitamin you should take to stay healthy. Too much of certain vitamins, such as vitamins A and D, can be harmful. Sometimes lots of vitamins are added to one pill or powder. The ancient Aztecs of Mexico made up a powder called spirulina, which is still made today.

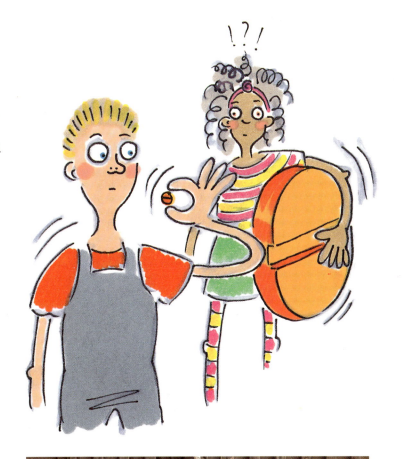

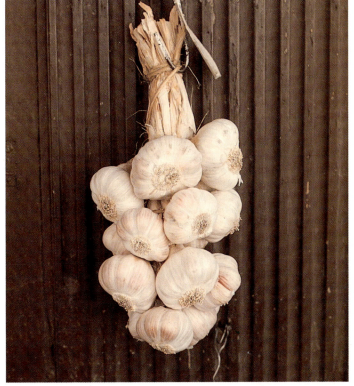

► *Garlic is good for your blood. It has been used for centuries to improve health.*

Vitamins and energy

Young people use up lots of energy. Vitamin B1 is lost through sweating and B2 is used up in hard exercise. These vitamins need to be replaced for your body to work well. The best way is to make sure that there are enough vitamins in your food.

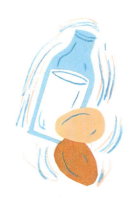

▼ *Vitamins are used up quickly in games and sports.*

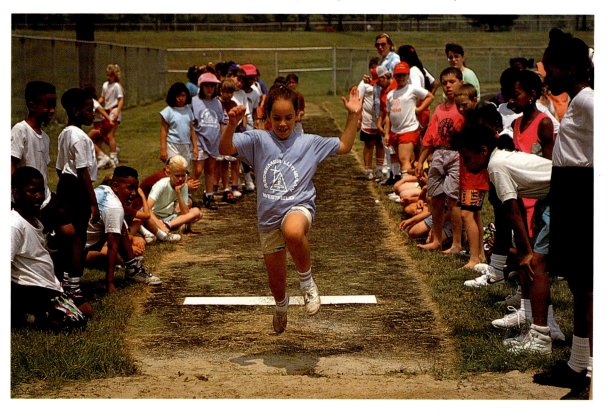

Looking for vitamins

This chart shows you where you can find the most important vitamins. Write down what you eat in one day and then check how healthy your diet is.

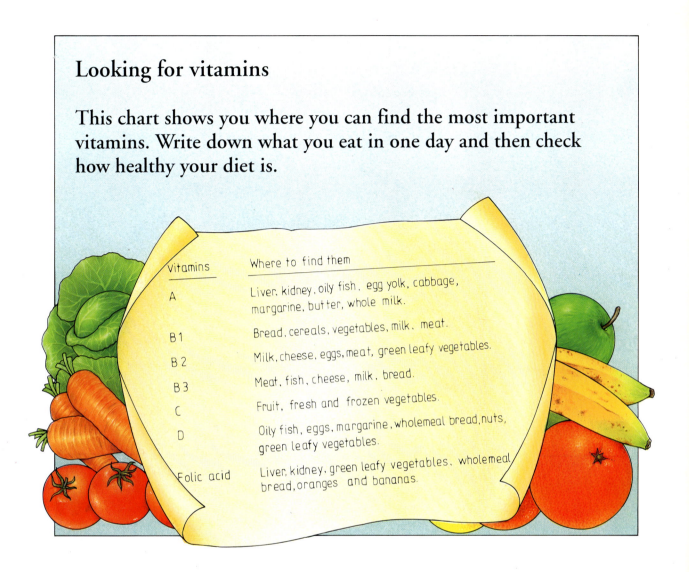

Vitamins	Where to find them
A	Liver, kidney, oily fish, egg yolk, cabbage, margarine, butter, whole milk.
B 1	Bread, cereals, vegetables, milk, meat.
B 2	Milk, cheese, eggs, meat, green leafy vegetables.
B 3	Meat, fish, cheese, milk, bread.
C	Fruit, fresh and frozen vegetables.
D	Oily fish, eggs, margarine, wholemeal bread, nuts, green leafy vegetables.
Folic acid	Liver, kidney, green leafy vegetables, wholemeal bread, oranges and bananas.

Some people need extra vitamins. Elderly people who eat less may need to take extra vitamins. Their bodies are slower at taking the vitamins out of food. Cigarette smokers destroy the vitamins in their bodies. The amount of vitamin C needed for one day is destroyed by just one cigarette!

Destroying vitamins

The longer food is left out in the light and the air, the fewer vitamins and minerals it will contain. Cooking food also destroys vitamins. Vitamin C is lost when fruit and vegetables are soaked and cooked in water. Steaming food keeps in more goodness, but uncooked fruit and vegetables are the best!

► *This girl is eating in a fast-food restaurant. Her food contains fewer vitamins and minerals than freshly made food.*

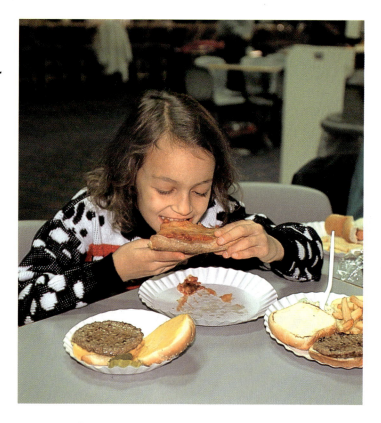

Healthy eating

Why not plan a healthy menu for a friend? Make sure that the meal contains as many vitamins and minerals as possible. Here is an example of a healthy lunch, to help you.

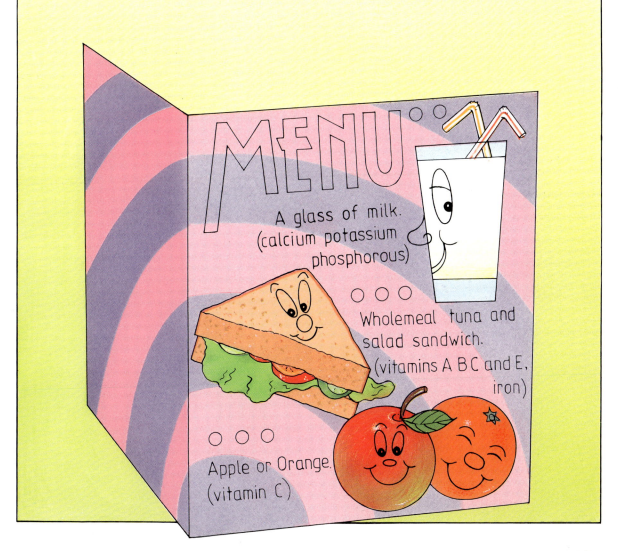

MENU

A glass of milk.
(calcium potassium phosphorous)

Wholemeal tuna and salad sandwich.
(vitamins A B C and E, iron)

Apple or Orange.
(vitamin C)

Glossary

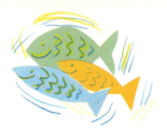

Aztecs   People who lived in Mexico in ancient times.

citrus fruit   A group name for lemons, limes, grapefruits and oranges.

fast food Food which is made in large amounts and sold to be eaten quickly.

husk   The outside covering of a seed.

pith   The soft white lining inside fruit such as oranges.

pulp   The soft flesh of a fruit. The pulp of an apple is the part you eat.

steaming   Cooking food in a container above steaming, boiling water. The hot steam cooks the food.

threshing   Beating ripe plants to separate the seeds from the stalks.

wheat germ   The seeds of the wheat plant.

yeast   An ingredient used in bread-making which helps the dough to rise.

Books to read

Diet   by Brian Ward (Franklin Watts, 1991)

Food Fun Book   by Rosemary Stanton (Hamlyn, 1988)

Fruit   by Miriam Moss (A & C Black, 1990)

Healthy Eating   by Wayne Jackman (Wayland, 1990)

Picture acknowledgements
Chapel Studio 8, 9, 23, 24; Bruce Coleman 6; Eye Ubiquitous 21; J.Greenberg 10, 26, 28; Tony Stone 5, 12, 14, 25; Zefa 7. The cover was photographed by Zul Mukhida and styled by Zoe Hargreaves.

Index

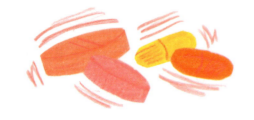

32